SPIRITUAL ENERGY HEALING

The New Healers Basic Guide For Healing
The Body & The Mind

Written By

Rev. Dr. Geraldine L. Johnson-Carter

*"Jesus was the greatest spiritual-energy healer ever!!!! Healing was a significant part of His ministry. He told us in John 14:12 that we who believe in Him will be able to perform the works that He would do and greater. All it takes is for us to **BELIEVE**!"*

Under no circumstances will any legal responsibility or blame be held against the publisher for any reparation, damages, or monetary loss due to the information herein, either directly or indirectly.

Respective authors own all copyrights not held by the publisher.

The information herein is offered for informational purposes solely, and is universal as so. The presentation of the information is without contract or any type of guarantee assurance.

The trademarks that are used are without any consent, and the publication of the trademark is without permission or backing by the trademark owner. All trademarks and brands within this book are for clarifying purposes only and are then owned by the owners themselves, not affiliated with this document.

Table of Contents

"Worship the Lord your GOD and his blessings will be on your food and water. I will take away sickness from among you." -Exodus 23:25

The world is not in need of a new religion, nor is the world in need of a new philosophy. What the world needs is healing and regeneration. The world needs people who, through devotion to God, are so filled with the Holy Spirit that they can be the instrument through which healing takes place.

Because healing is important to everyone, more and more spiritual healing is being discussed openly and practiced. It has been found that at some time or another, most of us will be in need of healing.

When we fall ill we find that a trip to the herbalist, homeopath and/or medical doctor will often get us back on the right track again. Sometimes, the illness will require more in-depth treatment and prescription drugs will be given to enable one to recover.

Or it might even be necessary to receive hospitalization for special intensive treatment. There is another form of treatment to consider when we fall ill and especially when traditional health care does not seem to work for us or has given up on us and that is Spiritual healing.

Quality health care is something that should be of interest to all of us, because good health is the right of all of us. Unfortunately, that doesn't often prove to be the case. Many people, for no apparent reason, seem to suffer varying health problems throughout their lives.

People often find that even when all physical, mental, moral or financial problems have been eliminated there will still be an inner unrest.

Many people also have often been found to not be at peace within themselves.

No one will ever be completely, fully and wholly satisfied within, even when there are good economic conditions until they find their inner relationship and communication with their Creator-God.

The harmony of humankind can only be achieved when he/she finds God, when he/she arrives at an inner communication with that which is greater than themselves. That is the real healing and lasting healing. That is the HEALING THE WORLD SEEKS.

Regardless of how much happiness you might find in your friends and family, when you retire at night you will still be ALONE. There is something within each of us that longs to go home that longs to live with our Creator God.

One must realize that until one establishes constant contact with the Source of one's existence there will be unhappiness, dissatisfaction, incompleteness, regardless of how much health or wealth is his/her lot.

Healing is finding an inner communication with something far greater than anything in the world. It is spiritually finding ourselves in GOD. When we find ourselves truly at peace, there is an inner glow, which comes to us with the realization that God is ALWAYS in us and with us.

God has promised to never leave us or forsake us. Once the presence and power of God is felt resting in us and we are at peace the body can resume its normal functions, and those functions are carried on by a power that is not our own.

Once the presence and power of God is felt in the body then the body begins to show forth perfect complete health, youth, vitality, and strength, which are all gifts from God. Spiritual healing is the touch of the spirit of God in our soul.

And when that touches us, it awakens us to a new dimension of life in a higher spiritual dimension. Some skeptics would argue that spiritual healing achieves only a reduction of stress and thus an enhancement of the body's natural defense mechanisms.

Others would suggest that hormones may be produced, which have an extremely beneficial effect on the function of organs and tissues, or that antibodies in the immune system are strengthened.

They may also suggest that spiritual healing merely seeks to reinforce the mental attitude of patients so that they feel better in themselves. All of these opinions may be true to a certain extent.

There have been many recorded examples of spiritual healing.

Spiritual healing relies on natural powers, and is something that has been known to the human race for many centuries. "Where the Spirit of the Lord is, there is liberty" 2 Corinthians 3:17. We are all seeking a way to find God. There is a motivating force within, a pull encouraging us to find God.

Man is not the healer God is the healer. God is a power, a presence something available above which is known to the human mind. We must develop in ourselves the "Practice of the Presence" until realization comes, followed by demonstration.

So it is when you have the experience of one first conscious realization of a transcendental Presence and Power of the something we call God, Spirit the Christ. There we can say with Paul, "I live, yet not I, but the Christ lives in me.

"I can of mine own self do nothing…the Father that dwells in me, He does the work." John 5:30. Sometimes one individual can show a measure of health, harmony, inner peace, joy, satisfaction, and abundance sufficient unto his/her needs, in that degree, that person is a light to the world.

And then become an inspiration for others to follow, the light which fills them with the same hope, the same ambition, and that same willingness to sacrifice just a few hours a day to the end that they may also know God.

Sometimes we are likely to forget what an influence the life of one man or woman can be. Once the Holy Spirit descends upon us and we are lifted up out of what we might call "this world" after that we are no longer attracted to the things of this world.

And from then on we can live within our own inner being with the Bible and its metaphysical writings and the company of those on the spiritual path. All the rest just drop away and become less important in our lives.

ILLUMINATION comes from seeing God and asking Him to open your heart and soul so that you can have a closer walk with Him. Now the ultimate salvation of the world through spiritual healing, will come through you and me.

Spiritual healing is therefore not a New Age treatment. And many forms of complementary healing are far from being new trends. Aromatherapy and reflexology for example, can be traced back to the Egyptian herbalist from pictures found on ancient caves.

Even with advances in modern medical research and improvements in the drugs available to us, there is still an acute need for spiritual healing. The end result of spiritual healing is an end to suffering!

We are all capable of helping to heal both each other and ourselves although some people seem to be naturally gifted healers. However, we can all develop our healing gifts and learn how to use them for the healer to heal thyself.

All healing of others begins with SELF HEALING. Learning to use our ability to heal properly may be one of the biggest single factors in improving our lives on this planet, both for the present and for the future.

Good health in an important component of a happy lifestyle. Poor health means that you are unable to do the things that you have done before with the same gusto and enthusiasm and small tasks that once required little thought become insurmountable obstacles.

Spiritual healing in some cases is not a cure all. It is not unusual for people to have spiritual healing and discover that an improvement in their condition is a slow process. Unfortunately, miracles don't often happen where someone is cured immediately.

For spiritual healing to be successful, it is important that the patient and the healer are attuned, not only to each other but also in alignment with the healing energies. If there is tension or stress the healing energies will not flow freely.

It takes many years of work and preparation to be an effective healer, and these things cannot be rushed. Healers need to have high standards, much is expected of them, and it is only fair that the help they give matches the expectations of their patients.

The first thing you should appreciate about spiritual healing is that it is not a miracle treatment, and it also may not provide a complete cure for an illness or medical condition, sometimes only a temporary aid.

Not everybody can be, wants to be or will be cured. And as one providing spiritual healing, you should realize from the outset that there is a wealth of difference between truly healing and curing.

In spiritual healing, which is basically the channeling of powers from our Creator (God) for the benefit of the patient concerned, there will be in most cases, an improvement in the condition being treated.

But how much improvement will depend on the individual, as well as how advanced the disease may be at the time of initial consultation. The secret of healing must inevitably be learned first that God is the true healer.

And second, that the nature of God is wisdom and the function of God is not only to create an image after His own image and His own likeness, but to maintain and sustain that image including all mankind, in a divine embrace of harmony, wholeness, completeness and perfection.

Unfortunately, many people turn to spiritual healing as a last resort, when their disease is well advanced and this often means that the healing provided cannot be effective. In such cases, the best that can be achieved may be a reduction in the pain and anxiety being experienced.

In an attempt to understand spiritual healing, many people that a spiritual healer is working with, will start to wonder where the power is originating from. Those people who believe in God may suggest that the healing power comes from God.

Those who do not believe in God will point to the Shaman's of many cultures, and suggest that the power comes from Nature or from spirits. What you as a healer need to reinforce is that regardless of where the power to heal originates, it exists and is something that we can tap in to.

There are many theories put forward by practitioners of spiritual healing, all attempting to explain what they do and how their healing works, but in truth, the answer is we really don't know. Some people will suggest that the healing treatment is only a matter of faith.

The power of the mind, can trigger or lengthen the illness. Those who understand about the seven chakra centers (energy centers) and the aura (energy field) which surrounds each person's physical body), can bring about improvement.

Because each cell in the body brings its own energy source much like a little battery. The chakras are energy centers, regulating the flow of energy throughout our body. If the chakras are out of balance, or if the energies are blocked, the basic life force will be slowed down.

The correct functioning and balancing of the chakras is reflected in our health and well being. Those healers who understand reflexology and acupuncture will be aware of the energy channels within the body, and how manipulation of these channels.

Tapping into these channels can bring about relaxation and relief of pain or reduction in symptom in various parts of the body. Healing power is inherent in all of us. And if we understand how to tap into it we can truly become healers.

If we try to heal under our own power we will feel depleted of our personal energy. Because we are transferring everything that we have to the other person and this can run ourselves down in the process.

Because spiritual healing taps into a power source other than our own personal energy system, we will not run into these problems. We can't explain how spiritual healing works all we understand is that it does work.

Spiritual healing is all about tapping into the power available to us to help us improve our health should we become ill. Fortunately for us the power we need to tap into to heal is there for us all the time.

Both the power without and the power within come from the same ultimate source. One is external to us the other is internal. Spiritual healing involves the transference of energy from an outer source into the body as a whole or to a specific area of the body to bring about healing.

It also involves regenerating energies already present within the cells of the body that may be impaired or reduced in efficiency. Sometimes this healing is carried out by personal touch or one to one healing treatments.

At other times, this treatment is carried out at a distance. Everyone goes through hardships in life. Illness is a dis-ease or lack of ease of parts of the body with the whole. What the healer is really trying to do is reintroduce energy back into the body.

We can do this by acting as a channel for that energy, so that the natural harmony and balance of the body can be restored, and it will no longer be at dis ease with itself. At the time of the treatment, the healers mind and the mind of the patient should be in harmony.

This is so the energy is able to transfer through to the patient at a deeper level than would occur otherwise. If you think positively and think well your health can be improved even if only marginally.

Negative thoughts and beliefs can, and do have a strong effect on health. Your body can run down easily by overworking your mind. It is important to always try as much as possible to live in a PEACEFUL and CALM state of existence.

It has been found that it will extend your life to live without worry and stress. Many illnesses are caused by inadequate diets combined with poor lifestyle habits and negative thinking. Try hard to not allow yourself to get to a state of anxiety and tension and you will be a lot healthier.

Continue to reinforce that there is a God and that God is LOVE and if you want to experience the grace of God it is necessary to be in the flow and align yourself with God and receive grace from God as it is now flowing, always has flowed and always will flow.

God is eternal, God is everywhere and it is true that what the Father has is "mine." God is the same yesterday, today and will also be tomorrow and the nature of GOD is to heal disease John 16:15.

It is also true that God works in and through individuals and practitioners to assist with Spiritual healing. Spiritual healing is about treating the body and mind as a unit, as healing affects body, mind and emotions.

If one part of the body is unwell, it will affect the whole person, and thus the whole body will be subject to the healing process, not just the part of the body causing problems. Spiritual healing does not confine itself to mere body parts.

It also encompasses the mental and emotional aspects of the person. Occasionally, in order to supplement the healing process special diets are suggested along with exercise. Good health can have a lot to do with a person's attitude, emotions and abilities to be positive.

Negativity is the state of being continuously anxious and worried. And this can have a detrimental effect on the body and make situations worse. A little anxiety and tension is good for us, and is necessary for the body to work effectively.

But all too often, we are subject to allowing a lot of stress and tension to affect us which in turn creates more anxieties, worries and depressions. It is also fair to say that a negative attitude from doctor's and other's can contribute to a general state of negativity for many patients.

RELAXATION on the part of the healer and the patient is necessary and important to successful healing. The healer must feel genuine compassion and love for the patient, and sincerely wish to see that person's health will improve.

The Spiritual healer must acknowledge God as the power who does the healing because if we acknowledge GOD, GOD will direct our path in the healing process. Spiritual healers do not tell their patient he or she is incurable.

Unfortunately, spiritual healing is often sought as a last resort when the body is already under attack from a disease which it cannot recover. But spiritual healing will at the very least, have a positive psychological effect to help the patient become relieved of their stress and tension.

Re-introduction of positive thoughts can completely reverse the downward spiral. It is possible to heal ourselves with spiritual healing. In fact, the body usually heals itself, even if we are not consciously aware of it.

The body has an immune system that fights off infections, viruses and diseases. Sometimes when our immune system's working well, we will not become infected with a cold or virus, while everybody around us will seem to be ill with coughs and colds.

We all develop cancerous cells at sometime in our lives. But normally a healthy immune system will spring into action and the diseased cells will be attacked and destroyed. Drugs have been developed that contain bacteria to strengthen the immune system and help fight against illness.

It is important to recognize that it has been found that some people do not want to be well because then they will not receive the attention and care they feel they have been lacking in their lives. (Spiritual healing will not work with people who want to be ill for whatever reason.)

Before your body can start to heal itself, you should be as relaxed as possible. Learn to meditate and to focus within, soothing music can help as well as a peaceful environment.

Meditation can bring about an altered state of consciousness.

Early spiritual and energy healers believed that there was a close link between the body and the mind. And that people had within themselves everything necessary to heal their mind and body. And that the only function they served was to help the person concerned discover this for themselves.

In meditation we are listening for the voice of God. We are not asking for anything other than more of God. Energy around and in us can be harnessed to activate self-healing through the power of love, breathing, relaxation and yoga.

Prana means breath, life force or an absolute energy, vitality and power. Prana is present in everything that exists in our lives. It enters our bodies when we are born and leaves our bodies when we die.

It flows through our bodies while we maintain good health in balance and undisturbed while we maintain good health. We cannot increase the amount of breath we have but we can reduce it significantly by lifestyle, our mental attitude and diet.

Once the balance or harmony is disturbed, our prana is also disturbed and ill health or dis ease results. Stress can bring about headaches, digestive problems and the illnesses that negatively influence our life force.

Prana being the life force or universal energy also has the power to heal, and once we find ourselves able to link with universal energy we can bring about our own healing and the healing of others. Certain areas of the world seem to have more power than others.

Hindus tend to believe that prana is more concentrated at the top of mountains and near running water. Throughout the day we come in contact with other people's energy and it reacts to our energy, as well as our energy reacts to theirs.

It is important at night to wash ourselves, to bathe or shower to rid ourselves of other people's energies and negative energies from our modern times such as electronic equipment etc. Washing our bodies is the easiest way to clear ourselves of negative energy on a daily basis.

Because water is a natural substance with its own natural energy, we can do a lot to restore our energy with a bath containing Epson salt. We can also use pleasant smelling essential oils, such as lavender and gentle music before we go to sleep to promote relaxation and remove negative energy.

Spiritual healing taps into the universal energy rather than the energy systems within each of us. I need to stress that tapping into our own energy systems will reduce its efficacy. And we will end up feeling run down and energy depleted.

How To Feel Chi Energy

Rub hands together to create an energy spark that can then be used to aid relaxation and help with the healing process. Try rubbing your hands together then place them immediately in front of your face and nose, close your eyes and breathe in the heat and chi energy produced.

You are helping to take this energy into your body, through your lungs and into your bloodstream. Take some deep cleansing breaths and this will help you and your patient with overall relaxation. You may wish to keep your eyes open.

And without focusing directly on to your hands, allow energy to be absorbed through your eyes in that this helps with eye strain or headaches. What we are doing is using the chi energy to revitalize us.

Let's look at love which is the greatest force we have at our disposal, should we choose to use it for the good of others and for ourselves. If there is tension in your life, you are blocking the power of love by creating blockages in your chi or energy systems.

To learn about healing we must first learn more about love for healing is love. If we sincerely want to heal others, we have to desire to deep down. We have to have a genuine love of that other person and really want to see them well. It takes unconditional love to heal.

It is important to demand nothing of others and do not expect anything in return. Some believe there is a psychological connection between anger and cancer-stating those with cancer are really nice people who find difficulty in showing their emotions, anger being one of those.

It is important to be open with emotions to heal. When the transformation begins it is a gradual process that will evolve over time. One session of spiritual healing will not provide a cure, if a cure can be achieved. Breathing and relaxation is necessary for healing.

Relaxation isn't just sitting down in a chair by the television. Relaxation is letting go of your inner tension and stresses, or the flight or fight reaction. When we are relaxed our brain waves activities change.

We are trying to achieve a state of well being which is an alpha state because when we are relaxed our breathing slows down. When we are totally asleep we are in a Theta state and in a deep sleep we enter a delta state.

The Auras - We know that the human body has energy running through it, which is similar to electricity. This energy radiates from the body. All living things whether plants or animals or human beings give off energy and this is called the aura.

Since ancient times people have believed in the existence of the aura, and it appears in the writings and art of many ancient cultures and civilizations. Most spiritual /energy healers will agree that the body has its own magnetic field known as the bio field.

It is important for anybody who wishes to carry out healing in any way to be familiar with the aura, and how it shows up to create problems in a person's health. So we must learn how to see the aura for ourselves.

To achieve a healthy aura we must have a proper diet, adequate sleep, reduction in stress and correct mental attitude. All are necessary to tap into the universal energies and apply the knowledge we have learned.

Proper breathing, the right environment, energy work, a low stress lifestyle, relaxation as well as consistent physical exercise is an extremely important component of a healthy and strong body and aura.

The Chakra Centers - chakras are spinning wheels of energy that rotate at various speeds for the whole of our lifetime. As the chakras spin, they radiate out the Universal Power to the glands to which they correspond, and also out into the aura.

The chakras are thought to play an important role in health, from both a physical standpoint and an emotional or spiritual standpoint as illness manifests itself not only in the aura but also in the chakras, through which the universal energy flows.

Each chakra center reacts to color and sound. If the chakra centers are unbalanced or blocked, illness or general debilities results, but this malaise works both ways, as our mental attitude can also affect the chakra centers.

The 7 Main Chakra Centers

The *First* Chakra is located at the base of the spine. This center is our link with the physical world. It absorbs energy from the planet and is able to "refine" this energy for use within our system.

This Chakra is concerned with issues related to our self-preservation, survival and security. The energies of the root Chakra impact on the body via the adrenal glands. They may also affect the functioning of the kidneys and the spine.

The *Second* Chakra is located at the sacral bones of the spine, below the navel, this center processes issues connected with our creativity, sexuality and the ability to play and express joy. The energies of the sacral or abdomen chakra are situated close to the genital organs and controls sexual urges.

They may also affect the organs of the body that include the uterus, kidneys, the heart, the lower digestive organs and lower back. When in a balanced state the sacral Chakra vibrates to the color orange.

The **Third** Chakra solar plexus chakra is located just below the diaphragm near the navel. It controls digestion and the endocrine system. This center processes all issues connected with the mind and emotions, personal power and sense of self.

Feelings of discomfort in this region may affect the diaphragm and our ability to breathe properly. The energies of this Chakra impact the body via the pancreas. It may also affect the gastric nerve, digestive system, pancreas, liver, gall bladder and stomach. When in a balanced state, the solar plexus Chakra vibrates to the color golden yellow.

The **Fourth** chakra is located in the center of the chest at the level of the heart. This Chakra processes all issues concerned with love, especially unconditional love and concern for others.

The energies of this Chakra impacts on the body via the thymus gland and can further affect the heart, lungs, chest, upper back and arms and controls respiration and emotions. When in a state of balance, the heart Chakra vibrates to the color emerald green.

The **Fifth** Chakra is located in the thyroid or throat. This Chakra processes all issues of communication, expression and judgment. The energies of this Chakra impact the body via the thyroid gland and can affect the neck, throat, ears, nose, mouth and teeth. In a state of balance, the throat Chakra vibrates to the color sky blue.

The **Sixth** or brow chakra is located in the middle of the forehead between the eyebrows. This Chakra processes all issues of psychic and intuitive awareness. Known since ancient times as the Third Eye.

The energies of this Chakra impact on the body via the pituitary gland and can further affect the nervous system, brain, face and eyes. When in a state of balance, the brow Chakra vibrates to the color indigo.

The **Seventh** Chakra is the crown Chakra and it is located at the top of the head. This Chakra processes all issues arising from our relationship with spiritual desires and is also connected with the cerebral functions and the rest of the body. When in a state of balance, the crown Chakra vibrates to the color purple or violet.

NOTE: The energies of a Chakra may also be detected at the back of the body as well as the front. The Universal Power enters the aura through the chakra at the top of the head, and works downward through the other chakras, each center using and changing the energy it receives according to the function that it governs.

The Root or base chakra influences kidney or bladder problem, problems with the process of elimination, obesity and with the lower back. Affected by fear, anger and sexual urge. Clear the blockages using white light –stimulate with red or orange.

The Spleen Chakra – influences digestive problems, reproductive problems, legs and feet. Affected by our sensitivities to others and those with lack of self-esteem or motivation will have a blockage here, feeling confused or restless. Clear blockages with orange. Stimulate using green, blue or violet.

The Solar Plexus Chakra – influences heart problems, nervous difficulties or skin problems, stomach or kidney problems. Those people who repress their feelings often have blockages here. Clear blockages using blue or violet. Stimulate the chakra using yellow.

The Heart Chakra – Immunity deficiency, circulation or breathing problems, also blood pressure or heart disease. Affected by anger and cleared by love. Clear blockages with indigo or red. Stimulate the chakra using green, rose or blue. It is said that when this chakra is open all others will come into alignment with it.

Throat Chakra – thyroid problems, lymphatic or oral problems, stiff neck, colds and flu, poor hearing, shoulders, arms and hands. Affected by lack of expression being allowed, stress, anxieties, fear and general negatives. Clear blockages with blue or violet. Also try mantras, prayer or soothing music. Stimulate the chakra using red.

Brow Chakra - migraine headaches, ear and eye problems, sinusitis. Also problems with the pituitary gland. Affected by fear, worry and doubts. Clear blockages with green. Stimulate the chakra using blue or indigo.

Crown Chakra – seasonal depression (SAD) depression or lack or mental clarity, boredom, confusion, brain problems. Affected by selfishness. Clear blockages with gold or indigo. Stimulate the chakra using white. NOTE: Energy or spiritual healing addresses the 'subtle energy body' that governs the physical body.

Working directly with the emotional, mental and spiritual dimensions of this energy body, the healer affects the healing and releases of blocked and distorted energy patterns, enabling the innate intelligence to operate freely, restoring physical, mental, emotional and spiritual health.

Truly a mind and body discipline spiritual/energy healing accelerates ones personal growth. Spiritual/Energy healing works in conjunction with and as an adjunct to medical and non-medical therapies.

As Humans are essentially electromagnetic beings, it makes perfect sense that the best possible modality for healing is energy/spiritual. That energy supports our life process in our physical, mental, emotional and spiritual bodies. This energy is our spiritual source of life.

This energy field acts as a bridge, a connection between the realm of pure spirit and the material world. It is both an indicator and regulator of the manner in which the life force is expressed in our worldly life.

If this energy field is clear, healthy and free from defects, we will likewise exhibit good health in all of its physical, emotional, mental and spiritual aspects. This is what it means when a person is in balance.

How To Provide Treatment For The Chakra's

For treating the chakras, open the treatment with prayer and end the treatment with prayer. Get to the alpha state and begin to visualize positive outcomes for seemingly difficult circumstances.

A positive mental attitude can help us feel better about ourselves. The Mind is the Builder! When we change our attitudes about our health we can change our health.

* Reduce stress and tension-reduce negativities
* Learn to be patient both with ourselves and with others
* Never be jealous or possessive
* Forgive
* No one is perfect so do not judge others
* Do not be hard on ourselves and we will in turn learn to not be hard on others

Achieve Healing By Using The Power Of The Mind

The power of the mind is a great thing. If we learn to use our minds to their fullest potential we can accomplish things that would previously have seemed impossible. Once we feel we can do something, we normally can unless of course, our expectations are ridiculous and totally unattainable to start off with.

#1. Set goals that we feel are attainable.

#2. Learn how to be positive.

#3. Learn how to visualize positive outcomes to situations.

We can do a lot to speed up the healing process and produce changes in our physical state by mind power alone. This mental attitude is all part and parcel of helping ourselves, as it is totally wrong to be reliant upon anybody else without being prepared to accept some of the responsibility ourselves.

Creative Visualization

Creative Visualization uses the power of imagination and the power of the mind.' The process is deciding what you really need and visualizing it and creating mind power so you get it. Relaxation is important to the process.

It has been suggested by noted spiritual healers that a combination of prayer, faith in God, a positive frame of mind and affirmations could produce a positive outcome when there is an illness or situation one would like to change.

There are some who believe that every thought you think creates your future. We are all capable of creating visual images. We do so every night when we dream. All we have to do is to create such visual images while we are still awake like (a day dream - positive day dreaming).

Paracelsus linked the power of the mind, or imagination, and the power to cause and cure illnesses. This is called the law of reverse effect. Matthew Manning carried out studies on cancer patients asking them to visualize, order and instruct their white blood cells.

The white blood cells are the body's own defense system, to become so active and strong that they overcome the disease. Other healers suggest using the imagination to visualize ships coming in and taking the disease out to sea or similar thoughts.

In many cases a remission of the disease is achieved, and in some cases the disease seems to disappear after using using these visualization techniques. This is the example showing the power of the mind on the body.

NOTE: The person has to feel comfortable with this technique. Suggest to the patient that their own energy system which can be linked to a gentle stream is carrying the disease out of the body and out to sea.

The patient must be willing to help themselves and alter their lifestyles, diet or whatever they can do to address the issue. The person is in charge and at the end of the day they are telling their bodies how to respond.

Healers can make suggestions to their patients, but nobody has the right to tell another person what to think or what to do. With creative visualization we are attempting to help the body help itself.

If when using creative visualization for better health, we think less of becoming totally well and think more of becoming a little better, our expectations change, become more in the realms of possibility, and more is achieved as a result.

Set small goals for the healing process and then review them on a daily basis. Either bringing them nearer if we need to, or when things are going well, this means moving them a little further away.

Affirmations

Affirmations express optimism like "Every day in every way, I'm getting better and better!" French psychologist and pharmacist Emile Coue suggested that this statement be repeated during relaxation at least 20 times to be effective.

The Power Of Prayer

We are all familiar with the concept of prayer. We might not all actively pray in the same way, but we all know of and are familiar with the concept of prayer. Even if you only think of prayer as a means of expressing your hopes and fears, the act of prayer, or focusing your attention on situations that concern you, is a good thing. Prayers do work.

Anybody can pray, anywhere, at anytime, alone or with other people. Prayer can be short or long, prayer can cover any distance so we can pray for people on the other side of the world, it can be personal or impersonal. Prayer is a very versatile thing. Prayers should be personal things, and should be offered from the heart to God.

What we are doing when we pray is asking for help and saying thanks for help given and that can be done any time and anywhere. When we pray we should believe that we are talking to someone close, someone whom we can trust. Repetition of something without thought is not truly prayer. The Bible tells us much about prayer.

It explains to us that we should never feel abandoned or anxious about anything and that praying will help us (Philippians 4). Pray at the start of a spiritual healing session and at the end of the treatment for the help received. Asking for continued healing should be done at every healing session.

Healing With Changes In Lifestyle And Diet

All healing starts with self healing. People must want to do something positive for themselves, and that starts with what a person feeds their body. Your body is like a machine, and it needs fuel to work. We provide that fuel in the form of food and drink.

Think carefully about your meals. Breakfast should be cooked cereal, yogurt and fresh fruit or hard boiled eggs for protein. Avoid things high in fat! Eat a lot of fresh fruit and vegetables. Drink water because it flushes the system of impurities.

Healing Ourselves With Unconditional Love

Live your life for you and don't live your life your life in any way through other people. Don't look for what you personally lack in someone else and expect they will make you a whole person. Truly love yourself unconditionally.

Find that missing link in yourself and develop yourself as a person, rather than trying to draw from them. Be truthful with yourself and others. Identify your shortcomings and work on them. Try to live a spiritual life, following perhaps the example of Jesus.

Healing Skills

Wash your hands under running water before you undertake any healing. Make sure that you are relaxed by taking deep breathes in through your nose, and then out through your mouth. Taking in deeply the Universal power of breath. Do this several times.

Do not diagnose. Ask your patient what the problem is, the symptoms and whether or not a doctor has been consulted. And if so, what the diagnosis was. Explain that you will be using the Universal Power and that you may be appropriately touching them.

Make suggestions on how they may alter their lifestyle, attitude but don't lecture them. Have the patient remove their shoes and sit in a chair. See if the patient wants to discuss the meditative state they entered into after the healing.

The patient needs to help him or herself as well as allowing you to help through using the Universal Power. Spiritual Healers should not charge people for healing. The motivation of healers should be to help other people, not to use other people's illness for their own personal gain.

Healers Pledge

"True healers will be taken care of by the universal energy. I am richly rewarded and abundant. I will always have enough for what I need."
(Affirm This Daily)

Tip: Try to spend money and time only on things that bring you ABSOLUTE JOY!

THANK YOU FOR READING!

If You Received Useful Tools In This Information, Please Give Me A 4-5 Star Rating!

This serves as a reward for an author. It takes hours and months, sometimes years of no pay to put together books for the purpose of sharing information you see as important to the world.

Please just take out a minute of your time and please leave a quick positive review. Thank you tremendously for taking out the time to read this information and knowledge.

If you really took this information seriously and you applied the key principles into your daily life, I KNOW you are seeing results.

So again, I thank you for your interest in learning and any investment in applied knowledge will always be a winning investment.

For More Books By

Rev. Dr. Geraldine L. Johnson-Carter
Visit:

amazon.com/author/
geraldinejohnsoncarter

www.ingramcontent.com/pod-product-compliance
Lightning Source LLC
Chambersburg PA
CBHW030527290526
45786CB00004B/1653